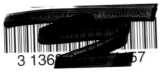
J
613   Giddens, Sandra.
              Making smart choices about food,
           nutrition, and lifestyle / Sandra
           Giddens. -- Rosen, c2008.

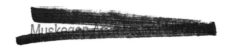

           I. Title.

making smart choices™

making smart choices about
food, nutrition, and lifestyle

Dr. Sandra Giddens and Dr. Owen Giddens

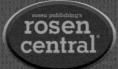

rosen publishing's
rosen central®

New York

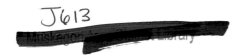

Published in 2008 by The Rosen Publishing Group, Inc.
29 East 21st Street, New York, NY 10010

Library of Congress Cataloging-in-Publication Data

Giddens, Sandra.
Making smart choices about food, nutrition, and lifestyle / Sandra Giddens and Owen Giddens.—1st ed.
   p. cm—(Making smart choices)
Includes bibliographical references.
ISBN-13: 978-1-4042-1389-0 (library binding)
1. Teenagers—Nutrition—Juvenile literature. 2. Children—Nutrition—Juvenile literature. 3. Health—Juvenile literature. I. Giddens, Owen. II. Title.
RJ235.G53 2008
613'.0433—dc22

2007032168

Manufactured in Malaysia

contents

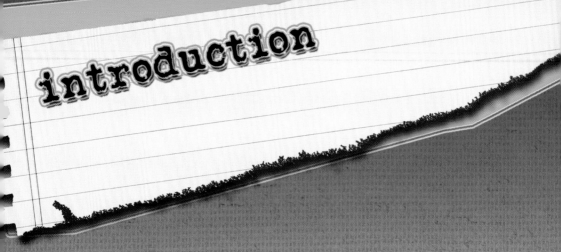

Every day, the media publishes headlines that read "Americans Getting Fatter," "Obesity on the Rise," and "On the Road to Diabetes." Advertisements urge consumers to "Try the new celebrity diet," "Lose weight instantly," "Explore this breakthrough technique in cosmetic surgery," and "Get a complete makeover."

Your parents, peers, teachers, religion, and, of course, the media all give you very strong messages on how to lead your life in terms of food, nutrition, and lifestyle. Despite this constant input, it is your responsibility alone to make choices that could affect you for a lifetime. You also have the freedom to change your choices along the way if you see that you are traveling a path that is obviously not right for you.

Remember, all choices have certain consequences, either good or bad. You can choose role models like Nicole Richie and Mary-Kate Olsen and aim to be unhealthily thin. Or you can continually take that second helping of cake and eat similar junk food all day. You can get a minimal amount of sleep and yet still convince yourself that you will function anyway. After school every day, you can either get involved in a physical activity or sit in front of the computer e-mailing your friends into the wee hours of the night. You can listen to your teachers who promote living a life being physically active, or you can be a telephone-talking couch potato, getting caught up on all the gossip, huffing and puffing as you travel back and forth to the fridge.

Everything you do affects your day-to-day living and general health. It is important for you to learn about your choices regarding what to eat, what nutrients foods contain, how much exercise you really require, and generally what is needed to feel healthy. It is vital that you feel good about yourself physically, mentally, and emotionally. If you are stuck in an unhealthy rut, you also need to know that you can alter your decisions and make changes at any time along the way.

chapter one

What Are Food, Nutrition, and Lifestyle?

You cannot live without food. Food is needed to give you energy. It is an essential part of family celebrations and religious festivities. Food is connected to entertainment, such as when you eat buttered pop-corn at the movies or hot dogs at baseball games. You cannot open a maga-zine or newspaper without seeing numerous articles and advertisements related to food and drink. When you walk through a shopping mall, you're bombarded with the far-reaching smells of the food court.

The variety of food is enormous, since we

Snacks may contribute up to one-third of your total daily caloric and nutrient needs. Irresponsible snack choices can lead to poor nutrition and weight gain.

live in a multicultural society. We also live in a world filled with fast-food restaurants that have engaging slogans and slick marketing that entice you to enter their doors. Food is everywhere, and you have countless choices of what to eat.

You are what you eat. To remain healthy, everyone requires a diet containing foods that contain the proper nutrients and vitamins. It is also essential that you eat enough food to be a healthy weight for your height. It is unhealthy to be either underweight or overweight.

Eating too many foods that are high in fat and sugar can make you overweight. Most food packaging has the ingredients labeled right on them. By reading the labels on food packaging, you can tell how much sugar, salt, vitamins, fiber, calories, protein, and carbohydrates you would be consuming. Consuming nutritious food does improve your emotional outlook, your general health, and even your performance in school.

What Is Nutrition?

Nutrition is a three-part process. First, food or drink is consumed. Second, the body breaks down what is consumed into nutrients. Third, the nutrients enter the bloodstream and travel to different parts of the body where they are needed to keep you healthy.

Foods contain different nutrients that help to keep your body functioning properly. Each of these nutrients has a distinct and important function. Nutrients can be categorized as either macronutrients or micronutrients.

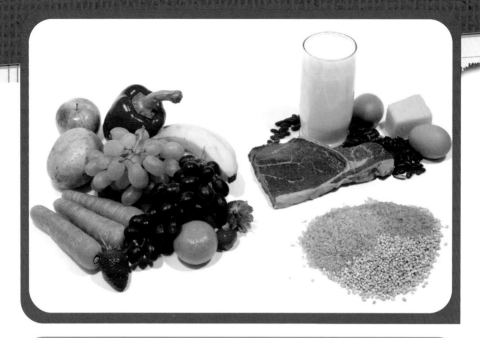

Maintaining a healthy diet keeps your body fit and energetic. Eating well-balanced meals provides your body with essential fats, proteins, carbohydrates, vitamins, and minerals.

Macronutrients are water, proteins, carbohydrates, and fats. Micronutrients are vitamins and minerals.

Water is the most abundant nutrient in your body, making up 50 to 70 percent of your weight. Protein is used to build and repair your body, including your hair and muscles. Carbohydrates and fats provide your body with energy. Vitamins and minerals are essential to maintaining your health. You require iron for your blood, calcium for your bones, and vitamin A for your eyes. Vitamin C keeps your skin healthy and helps in fighting illnesses. Choosing a diet that is low in fat and abundant in grain products, vegetables, and fruits is crucial to your health. Such good nutrition involves eating a variety of healthy foods and balancing your intake with physical activity.

The food pyramid shows the food groups and teaches you the proper way to eat. In the food pyramid category, choices such as pasta, bread, bagels, tortillas, rice, and cereal are all included.

What Is Health?

The World Health Organization (WHO) defines health as "a state of complete physical, mental and social well-being, and not merely the absence of disease or infirmity."

Everyone aims to be healthy. Eating right, sleeping well, exercising often, and not experiencing too much stress contribute to your well-being. Being well means taking good care of yourself from the outside to the inside. On the outside, it is vital to keep yourself clean and well groomed, and on the inside, it is important to feel emotionally well.

Food provides your body with energy. Exercise uses up this energy. In order to maintain a healthy weight, the amount of calories you consume should equal the amount of calories you burn. Exercise burns fat, builds muscles, and contributes to overall good health.

Adolescence is a busy time for you because your life fills up with school, sports, peers, family functions, and other social activities. It is also a time when your body is changing rapidly, and you are going through a series of growth spurts. Many girls naturally gain weight during puberty, as their hips widen and their body fat increases. Boys also have their growth spurts at different times and may feel troubled if they are not lean and muscular.

Adolescent bodies are growing into adult bodies and therefore need proper nutrition to further this process along. Regular checkups from your family doctor and dentist are also needed to keep up your good health. Yet, for many, adolescence is the time when they eat erratically and fill up on junk foods. Teens also tend to spend a lot of their time on cell phones and in front of

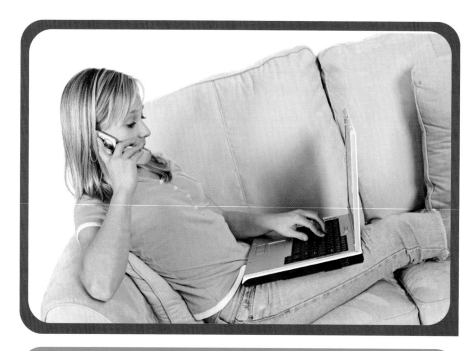

As part of the Internet generation, we can communicate with other people without leaving the couch. This convenience sometimes keeps us from getting the exercise we need.

the computer and television. They forget about the importance of exercise.

Influential Factors

The media are a major influence on the American lifestyle. Often, the media give mixed messages. They show excessively thin models and movie stars, which gives the underlying message that in order to be beautiful and successful, you have to be underweight. On the flip side, the media can be beneficial by warning that you may be at risk for diabetes and heart disease if you are struggling with obesity.

There are huge ads for diets and weight loss pills. At the same time, there is a rise in obesity, especially among children, who are bombarded with television ads promoting sugary cereals and junk food. This is the age when they are most likely to be influenced by these commercials.

Television gives the false impression that in order to be beautiful and happy, you need to be thin. There are makeover shows where the person comes in looking ordinary and, after undergoing thousands of dollars' worth of plastic surgery, he or she emerges looking beautiful. The final clip of these shows is of the person's family and friends applauding the transformation. Again, the message is that you have to change your appearance to get acceptance and happiness in life.

Dan Rather reported in a *48 Hours* documentary special that nearly 50 percent of all thirteen-year-old girls say they don't like how they look. By the age of eighteen, it's up to 80 percent. That is a disturbing phenomenon, as it means that for every ten girls, eight do not like how they look. If girls are so unhappy about their looks, it is needless to say that many are resorting to drastic measures like turning to cosmetic surgery, diet pills, and yo-yo dieting. One in five high school girls surveyed in Minneapolis admitted to using diet pills or laxatives, vomiting, or skipping meals altogether in order to become or stay thin. Now, boys are also fixated on their looks as well. They want to look buff like their role models, who tend to be professional athletes and movie stars. Boys, too, are beginning to be drawn to detrimental practices such as taking steroids and crash dieting.

Health Habits

You initially learn eating habits at home. But in our society of instant gratification, there has been more emphasis placed on buying fast and processed foods, such as frozen dinners, than on sitting down for lovingly prepared, wholesome meals at home. Also, with working parents, many families have staggered meals not eaten together as a family. The food for their kids is usually fast foods that are more convenient but are higher in fat.

Today, the cheaper foods, which are not necessarily nutritious, are becoming the norm. Fast-food companies have bought in to the idea that the bigger the portions, the better their business will be. As a result, consumers end up overweight. Another factor is the electronic generation. People spend hours and hours on the computer. Exercise

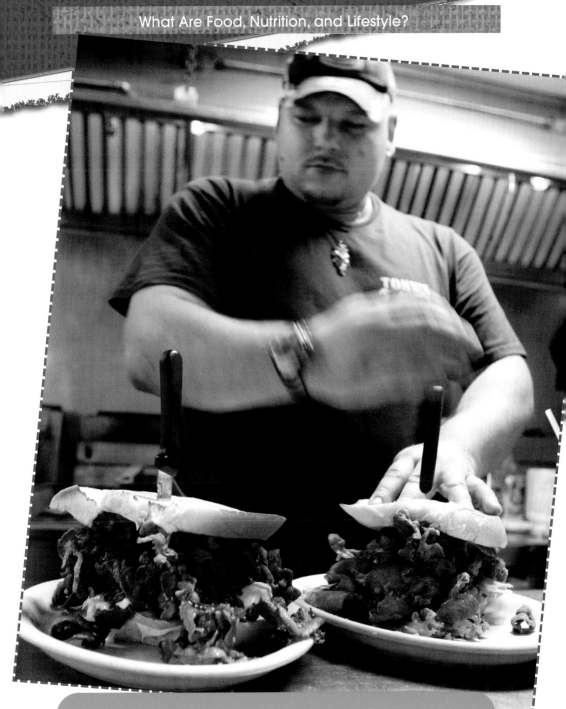

It is always about the food choices you make. Eating supersize sandwiches will only lead to a supersize you!

becomes something to fit in between computer time, if at all.

Making the Right Choice

With so many temptations out there, how do you make the right choices? For instance, your mother packs your lunch every day. It is filled with nutritional foods. You look around and see that a lot of your friends are ditching their healthy lunches and filling up on soft drinks and french fries. Do you throw away your lunch, too?

If you repeatedly throw away your lunch and eat junk food instead, your health will suffer. You know you need nutritional items in order to have energy and concentrate in school. If you throw away your lunch only this one time, no one will know or care, right? But if you are constantly throwing it away, will you be able to tell your mother to not bother making you lunch?

Do you feel better after you eat junk food? Do you think that eating non-nutritious foods helps you fit in with the more popular kids? If you start on a diet of junk food, will you eventually regret it? Can you limit yourself to only occasionally consuming soft drinks and french fries? Each decision you make leads you to another choice.

Teens have the freedom to make personal choices. Many are eating out more than their parents did when they were growing up. For lunch, they either visit fast-food restaurants or purchase food from school vending machines, which usually sell items like chocolate bars, chips, and soda. It is difficult to expect teens to brown-bag

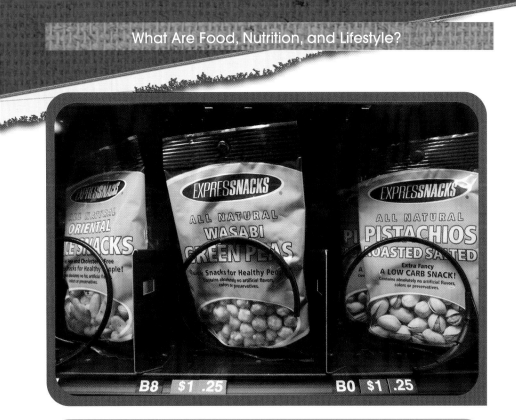

Most vending machines sell foods that have little or no nutritional value. If you look hard enough, though, you can find nutritious options such as nuts and dried fruits and vegetables.

their lunch every day, eating carrot sticks while many of their buddies go out for fast food.

Now may be the time to look at making better choices when you are in these situations. At many fast-food restaurants now, there are salad, grilled chicken, and fish options. At schools, there are vending machines that sell bottled water and bags of almonds, dried fruit, or trail mix. It is up to you to make the right choices about your diet and health.

chapter two
Your Choices About Food, Nutrition, and Lifestyle

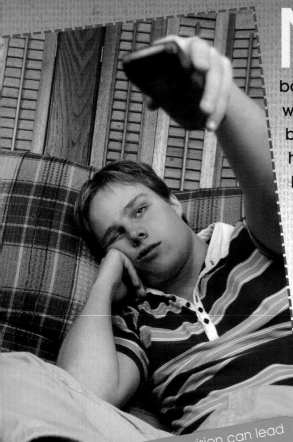

Watching too much television can lead to weight gain since you are less active and tend to eat high-fat snacks while watching.

Not all healthy teens look the same. For example, girls and boys have different healthy weight ranges because their bodies are different. Girls have more fat tissue, and boys have more muscle tissue. Since muscle weighs more than fat, a boy will usually weigh more than the girl of the same height. If you weigh too little or too much, then you may be at risk for health complications.

According to the 2006 *Journal of the American Medical Association,* the number of young people who are over-weight is increasing in

America. About 20 percent of U.S. teens are overweight, and obese teens tend to grow into obese adults.

Why this is has mainly to do with the choices people make in their lives. Many teens take a bus or car to school instead of walking. They sit in front of a computer or television screen for hours. According to Mary Turck, author of *Healthy Eating for Weight Management*, weight tends to increase with television watching. Children who watch fewer than two hours of television a day tend to weigh less than those who watch four or more hours. Typically, children plunk themselves in front of the television or computer screen for much more than four hours each night. Every time you sprawl in front of the television, your metabolism slows to a crawl. The average teen now spends almost thirty hours a week in front of the television, while eating high-fat snacks.

A lot of teens eat fast-food meals, which contain too much fat, salt, and sugar. To make things worse, these meals are often "super-sized." The combination of increased fast-food intake and less physical exercise leads teens to become overweight or even obese. There are many health risks for those who are obese. Some of these risks are:

- Diabetes
- Heart disease
- High cholesterol
- High blood pressure
- Breathing problems
- Sleeping problems

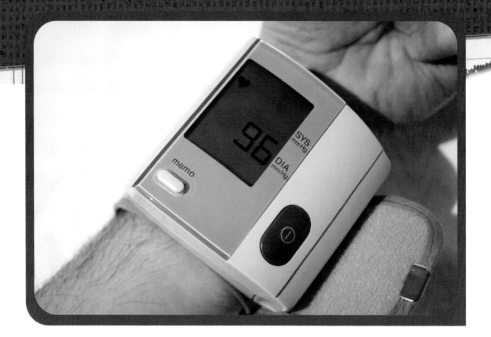

Up to 10 percent of teens may have high blood pressure as a result of being overweight or poor nutrition. High blood pressure raises their risk for heart disease and stroke in adulthood.

- Digestion problems
- Emotional problems

Reading about these health risks may scare you, but it still may be hard for you to resist having that extra helping at supper, eating the additional slice of cake for dessert, and drinking more than four sodas a day.

Eating Disorders

As you grow up, you start making your own choices on how to live your life. You can choose to be influenced by others, or you can choose to come to your own decisions wisely. One problem that has affected teens, especially girls, is that they feel the need to diet and be thin. If they're thin, they'll be more attractive to themselves and to others. They feel that their whole self-esteem rests on how they look.

Many teens going on a diet believe that being thinner will in fact improve their overall lives. There are many teens that start dieting and find that they cannot stop. They end up developing eating disorders. Three eating disorders are anorexia, bulimia nervosa, and binge-eating.

Anorexia is a condition in which a person severely restricts his or her food intake and loses a drastic amount of weight as a result. People with anorexia are obsessed with being thin. They don't want to eat because they are afraid of gaining weight. They may constantly worry about how many calories they take in or how much fat is in their food. They may take diet pills, laxatives, or water pills to continue to lose weight. In addition, they may exercise too much.

Anorexics think they are fat even when they are extremely thin. People with anorexia may get so thin that they become sick and have to be hospitalized.

With bulimia nervosa, the person eats a lot of food at once, or binges, and then vomits or uses laxatives to get rid of, or purge, the food. Some bulimics will overexercise after they binge-eat so that they do not gain any weight back. Others use water pills or diuretics, laxatives, and/or diet pills to control their weight. They often try to hide their bingeing and purging habits from other people, including

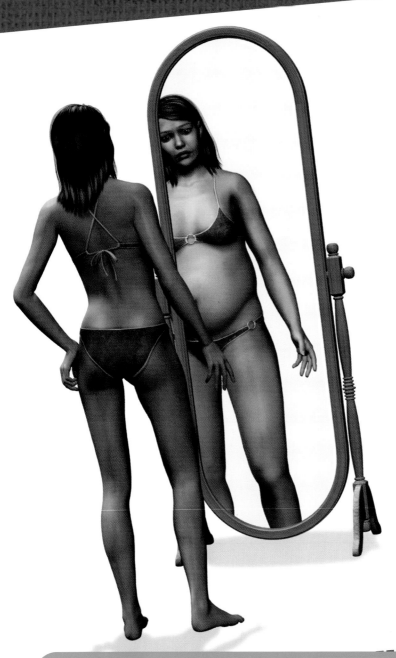

Body image is how you perceive your body independent of reality. Anorexics and bulimics believe they are overweight despite how thin their bodies truly are.

friends and family members. They also may hide food for their binges. Bulimics can be close to a normal weight, but their weight may go up and down.

Anorexia and bulimia are more prevalent among girls. However, an equal number of girls and boys suffer from binge-eating. Dieting is not a disorder in and of itself, but left unsupervised it can be a first step toward developing an eating disorder.

Staying Healthy

Becoming healthy and staying that way takes work. One important aspect of good health is proper hygiene. Showering or taking a bath keeps your body free of germs and helps prevent you from getting sick.

Your face in particular needs to be kept clean. Acne can begin during puberty, thanks to hormones, and persist well into the teen—or even adult—years. It is essential to keep your face and skin clean at all times.

Hand washing is vital in order to keep potentially harmful germs at bay. Whenever you have a cold, you run the risk of infecting others. So, always cover your mouth when you cough or sneeze, and be sure to wash your hands. If you have a body or tongue piercing, keep the area as sterile as possible.

The media has a field day with advertising products to keep you clean. There are numerous ads for soap, shampoo, detergents, and deodorants in magazines and newspapers and on television and billboards. The message is clear: to be healthy, be clean.

When you go to the doctor's office for a routine checkup, the doctor will check your height, weight, eyes, ears, throat, and blood pressure. You may even be asked for a urine sample. When talking with your doctor, the answers you give will determine whether the doctor needs to do additional tests.

For example, if you have trouble breathing, you may require a chest X-ray. When checking your blood pressure, the doctor wants to make sure that it is within the normal range. The doctor may also talk to you about your future risk of diabetes, heart disease, or osteoporosis.

If you have been feeling unwell, or have been too afraid to describe your symptoms to your doctor, you may be putting yourself at risk. Maybe you are feeling weak and all you require is more iron in your diet. Those headaches could be from eyestrain and you may need a new eyeglass prescription. Or perhaps you truly need to be referred to a specialist for further investigation. It is your body, your health, and your choice to keep it functioning to its maximum level.

Factors to Think About

Healthy living is a matter of choice. There is enough information that suggests eating right, getting enough exercise, and having a good mental outlook contribute to a healthy lifestyle. Not skipping meals like breakfast will help your body refuel. Snacks can consist of cheese and crackers, a piece of fruit, or yogurt. Some seemingly nutritious snacks are actually loaded with salt, sugar, and

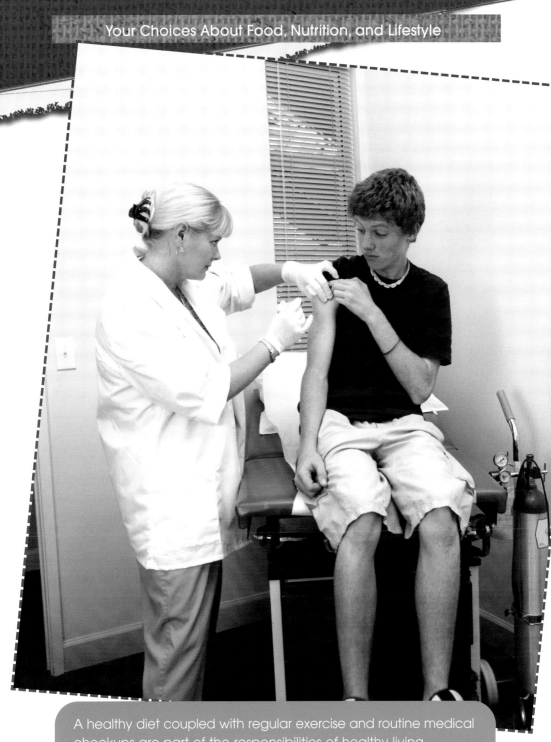

A healthy diet coupled with regular exercise and routine medical checkups are part of the responsibilities of healthy living.

calories. For example, some energy bars offer little nutritional value as they are loaded with salt and sugar. Fruit drinks also can be filled with sugar and contain few nutrients. Again, read the labels on foods to understand what you are consuming.

Healthy eating does not mean you cannot have the occasional piece of chocolate or bag of chips. If you are eating proper meals on a regular basis, you do not have to feel guilty for indulging in an unhealthy snack once in a while. It is all about moderation and reducing excess calories.

Your choices are that you can eat well-balanced meals or fill up on junk food. You can follow a daily exercise regimen or have a sedentary lifestyle. You can maintain good health by sleeping well, eating nutritiously, showering once a day, and getting regular checkups from your doctor and dentist. It's all up to you. Make decisions not based on impulse, the media, or the jealousy of others, but on correct knowledge and the desire to be as healthy as possible.

People with type 2 diabetes do not produce enough insulin. This form of diabetes tends to occur in overweight people. If the spread of this condition continues at today's rate, the number of Americans affected will increase to 22 million by 2025.

Although type 2 diabetes is partly genetic, it can be prevented or delayed. The key to doing this is to lead a healthy lifestyle. It means that you have to eat right. Do not overindulge in junk food such as sodas, doughnuts, and candy. Eat whole grains, rather than refined grains like white bread. Limit your

Diabetes is a disease of epidemic proportions in America. The good thing is that the risk for getting diabetes can be lowered by choosing a healthy lifestyle.

visits to fast-food restaurants. Try to avoid fried foods. Spend less than two hours a day in front of the computer or television. Exercise more.

If you are overweight, you may need the help of a dietician. Smoking and alcohol consumption put you at risk, too. Stay lean and stay active. Talk to your doctor about other ways to keep yourself from getting type 2 diabetes. After all, once you have type 2 diabetes, you are more susceptible to other health problems.

Osteoporosis

Osteoporosis is a bone disease that develops slowly, usually in females, and tends to be caused by genetics and too little calcium in the diet. When you have osteoporosis, your bones become so fragile that they can break. The condition also leads to shortened height and an increased chance of a hunched back because of collapsing spinal bones.

Calcium is vital for your body, as it makes your bones strong. During the teen years, bones develop quickly and store calcium so that you will have it later in life. If the amount of calcium stored in your bones is inadequate because you failed to eat a proper diet when you were young, your bones may become brittle and break in your old age.

Can osteoporosis be prevented? Do I have a choice? There are always going to be some risk factors, but if you include calcium in your diet (approximately 1,300 milligrams

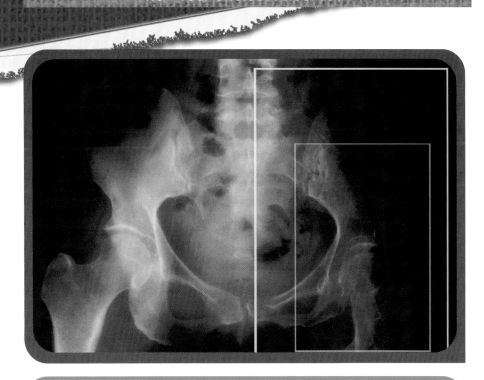

Osteoporosis causes weakened bones because of a lack of calcium. One way to prevent osteoporosis is to make sure you have calcium in your diet every day.

per day), get plenty of exercise, and do not smoke, then you will be farther ahead.

The Risks of Fad Diets

You have been reading this month's teen magazine, and it announces the latest fad diet that all the celebrities are supposedly on. It looks so easy.

People love to try all kinds of diets to lose weight, especially before big events like weddings and parties. There is the popular cabbage soup diet, the banana

27

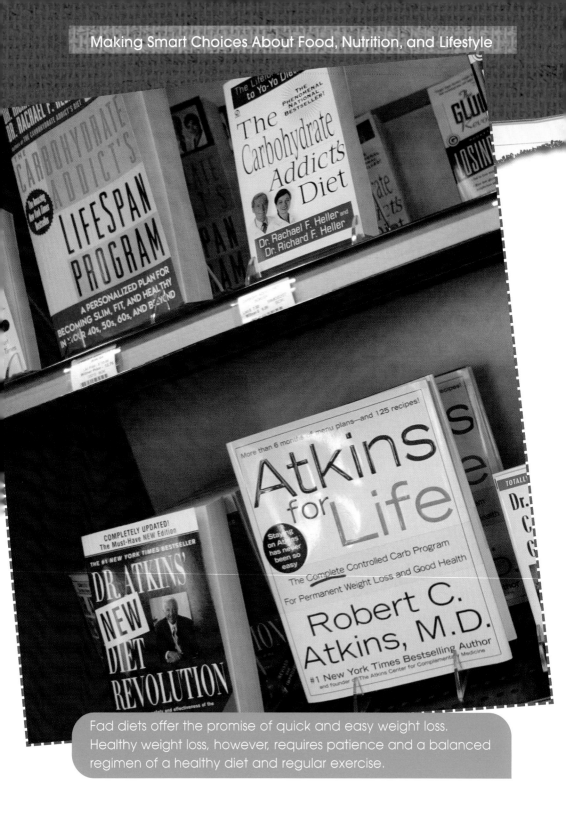

Fad diets offer the promise of quick and easy weight loss. Healthy weight loss, however, requires patience and a balanced regimen of a healthy diet and regular exercise.

diet, the high-protein diet, the fasting diet, and the body-cleansing diet, just to name a few.

There are diets that come with weigh-ins every week, vitamin shots, specially prepared foods, and calorie counters. There is a whole industry out there of diet foods and drinks, but many are not nutritionally sound.

Fad diets may be popular, but there are things wrong with them. One is that many are not nutritionally based. They prevent you from getting the calories and nutrients that you need to be healthy and for your bones to grow.

Another problem is that fad diets work in the short term, and the weight comes back quickly once you go off them. Many depend on water loss for quick results, and eventually, your body regains the water weight. Fad diets rarely provide long-lasting weight loss.

If you decide to go on a fad diet, there is always the fear that you will get involved in yo-yo dieting. That is when you go through a cycle of dieting, losing weight, not dieting, gaining the weight back, dieting again, and so on. For feedback, keep a journal of what you eat. Write down everything that passes your lips for a full week, as well as when you eat. Count how many calories you are consuming. The results may be surprising, but it will show you where you need to cut down.

It is always your choice to start a fad diet. If you do not like it, you can make the decision to stop it at any time. But if you start the diet and continue it, you could run the risk of getting sick. If you really need to diet, then going to a doctor or nutritionist for advice is the best way to go.

You could ignore the fad diets while flipping through teen magazines. The choice is yours to make.

Fats

Although all types of fat have the same amount of calories, some are more harmful to your health than others. Two of the most harmful fats are saturated fats and trans fats. Both can increase a person's risk of heart disease. Products including trans fats include many teen favorites: cookies and other baked goods, crackers, potato chips, tortilla chips, corn chips, energy bars, and french fries.

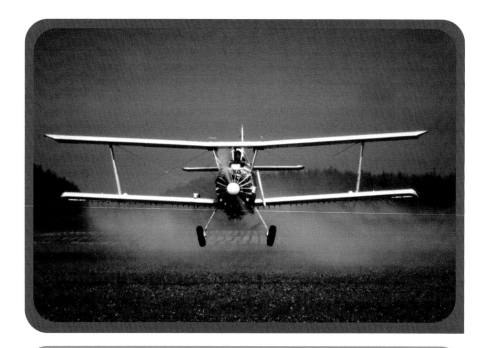

Food safety is not just about fats and cholesterol. Many people believe that pesticides sprayed on fruits and vegetables pose a health risk, so make sure you wash your foods before eating them.

Fortunately, some food companies are listening to the concerns of health-conscious consumers and, as a result, are removing trans fats from their products.

Cholesterol and Heart Disease

Heart disease continues to be the number-one cause of death in the United States. Teens usually do not show symptoms of heart disease, but the silent buildup of plaque or fatty deposits in the arteries can start in childhood and affect you later in life. Too much cholesterol in the body can lead to heart disease.

Being obese or diabetic, getting little or no exercise, smoking, and having high blood pressure all increase your chance of getting heart disease. If the disease is already prevalent among your immediate family, and you have one or more of the risk factors, then you need to be closely monitored by a doctor. Healthy living means being physically active and avoiding foods that are high in cholesterol, saturated fats, and trans fats.

Are you making the right choices for your health?

31

chapter four

Steps to a Healthy Lifestyle

The proverb "An ounce of prevention is worth a pound of cure" can apply to healthy living. It may be difficult to realize at your age what you do to your body now can affect you as an adult. It's hard to fathom that all those double cheeseburgers and french fries you are eating now can lead to health problems like diabetes, high cholesterol, and heart disease. How do you make the right choices?

It is important to have a realistic image of yourself. There is no single ideal and no perfect body. The right weight for one person can be

By maintaining a healthy diet, you can keep the pounds off and look and feel good both inside and out.

different for another. The doctor can help set the right goals for your body mass index and weight based on your age, height, genetics, and general health. Resist quick fixes like fad diets, as they can be detrimental. Weight-loss or diet pills can be dangerous, too. Losing weight and keeping it off are all about lifestyle choices. Always seek help from a doctor or nutritionist.

Watch What You Eat

Eat healthy quantities of food. It is far better to not "super-size" your meals. Recognize when you have hunger pains

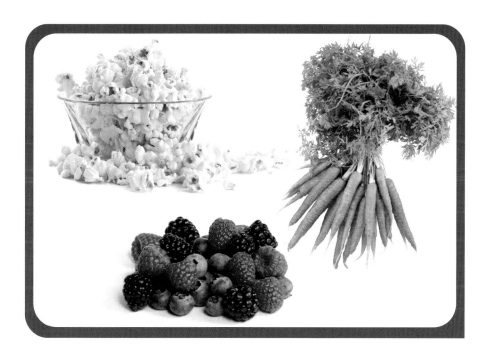

Evenings can be a tempting time to indulge in sugary, fatty snacks. Instead, choose healthier foods to satisfy your hunger. Carrots, berries, or air-popped popcorn can do the trick.

33

and when you are full. Sometimes, it's better to share a meal with your friend so you both can reduce your food intake. Try not to eat frequently at fast-food restaurants. When you do go, remember that burgers and fries contain about 1,300 calories, half the normal calorie intake for one day. Substituting a salad can reduce the calorie intake.

Watch what you drink. The calories in soft drinks, fruit juices, and other beverages can really add up. The average twelve-ounce can of soda has 150 calories and 10 teaspoons of sugar. A lot of specialty coffees are filled with sugar. Water is still one of your best choices. Choosing water instead of a sugary soda or fattening milkshake can make a huge difference.

Add more fruits and vegetables to your meals, or eat them alone as snacks. Other healthy snacks include low-fat yogurt, pretzels, graham crackers, air-popped popcorn, and string cheese.

It is important that you eat nutritiously. Look at ingredients on food packaging. Make sure you are getting enough calcium, protein, and vitamins. Check the food pyramid to see if you are eating properly. Practice good hygiene. See your doctor and dentist for regular checkups. These are all ways to take good care of your body.

Exercise

Another way to take good care of your body is to exercise. It has been said over and over again that regular exercise can improve your health, as it lessens your chances of getting heart disease, high blood pressure, and diabetes.

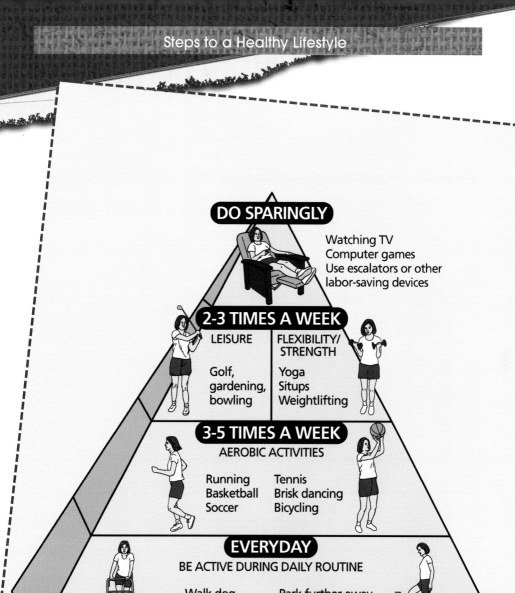

DO SPARINGLY

Watching TV
Computer games
Use escalators or other
labor-saving devices

2-3 TIMES A WEEK

LEISURE	FLEXIBILITY/ STRENGTH
Golf, gardening, bowling	Yoga Situps Weightlifting

3-5 TIMES A WEEK
AEROBIC ACTIVITIES

Running	Tennis
Basketball	Brisk dancing
Soccer	Bicycling

EVERYDAY
BE ACTIVE DURING DAILY ROUTINE

Walk dog	Park further away
Take stairs	Clean house
Do yardwork	Wash & wax car

Here is a simple guide to promote steps for a healthy, energetic lifestyle. By following this guide, you'll be maintaining a healthy exercise routine.

Exercise is also excellent for your emotional well-being, since it reduces feelings of depression, anxiety, and stress. Try doing about fifteen to thirty minutes of physical activity every day. If you can't do thirty minutes at once, split it up to three ten-minute periods. Do some weight training to help you improve your strength and build muscle. Find fun activities that you enjoy, like swimming, in-line skating, dancing, or biking.

Work with Your Family

You may need to advocate for your entire family to change their diet and exercise habits. Eat at least one meal together. Try nutritious recipes. Encourage your family to eat more fruits and vegetables. Do not stock up on junk food when grocery shopping. Do not snack while watching television. This helps to reduce mindless eating.

Introduce bicycling, hiking, walking, tennis, and other exercise that will benefit everyone.

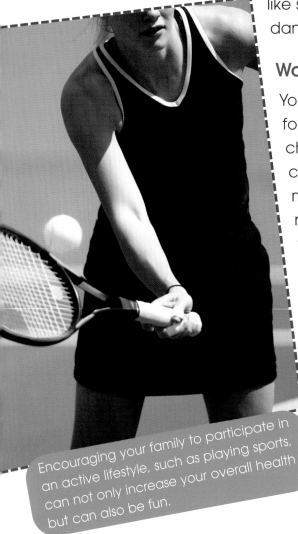

Encouraging your family to participate in an active lifestyle, such as playing sports, can not only increase your overall health but can also be fun.

Does anyone in your family have diabetes, heart disease, high blood pressure, or osteoporosis? If the answer is yes, then consult your family doctor before embarking on a group exercise regimen.

You Are on Your Way

Eating properly and exercising routinely can be hard work, but the benefits are more than worth it. Begin with small steps. If you believe that you can do it, then you are well on your way to having a healthy life.

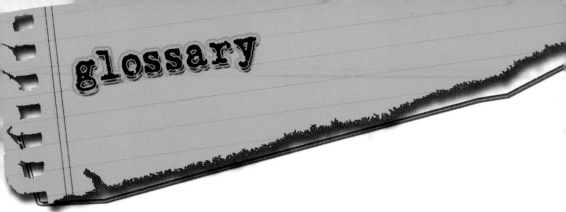

body image The way you perceive your body.

body mass index (BMI) A measurement designed to show whether a person is underweight, normal weight, or overweight. It is calculated from a person's weight and height.

calorie A measurement of the amount of energy that a food supplies.

carbohydrate A nutrient that provides energy; sugars and starches are carbohydrates.

diabetes A disease that prevents the body from being able to control the amount of sugar in the blood.

diuretic A chemical that stimulates the body to rid itself of fluids by urination; also known as a water pill.

eating disorder An unhealthy, out-of-control attitude toward weight, body image, food, and eating habits.

fad diet A popular eating plan for losing weight.

fat A nutrient that provides energy and is stored in the body.

metabolism A body process that breaks down food and turns it into energy.

nutrients The materials in food that your body needs to grow, have energy, and stay healthy.

obesity The condition of being more than 20 percent over a healthy weight.

puberty When a person matures from child to adult; this period of rapid development is set off by hormones.

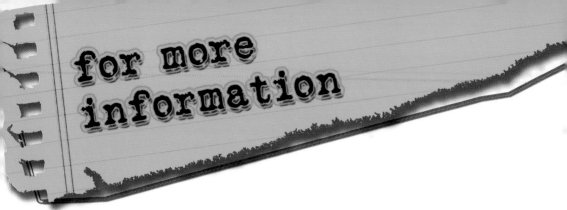

American Dietetic Association (ADA)
216 West Jackson Boulevard
Chicago, IL 60606-6995
(800) 366-1655
Web site: http://www.eatright.org
ADA serves the public by promoting optimal nutrition,
   health, and well-being. ADA members are the nation's
   food and nutrition experts, translating the science of
   nutrition into practical solutions for healthy living.

Anorexia Nervosa and Associated Disorders (ANAD)
109-2040 West 12th Avenue
Vancouver, BC V6J 2G2
Canada
(604) 739-2070
Web site: http://www.anad.org
ANAD is a nonprofit corporation that seeks to alleviate
   the problems of eating disorders, especially anorexia
   and bulimia. It strives to educate the public and
   healthcare professionals about illnesses related to
   eating disorders and the methods of treatment.

Health Canada
Health Promotions and Programs Branch
Nutrition and Healthy Eating Program
Jeanne Nance Building, Tunney's Pasture
Ottawa, ON K1A 1B4
Canada
Web site: http://www.hc-sc.gc.ca
Health Canada gives information from the latest recalls
    to the latest headlines having to do with health and
    nutrition in Canada.

National Association to Advance Fat Acceptance (NAAFA)
P.O. Box 188620
Sacramento, CA 95818
(800) 442-1214
Web site: http://www.naafa.org
NAAFA is a nonprofit human rights organization dedicated
    to improving the quality of life for fat people. It works to
    end discrimination based on body size and provide fat
    people with tools for self-empowerment through public
    education, advocacy, and member support.

National Eating Disorders Association (NEDA)
603 Stewart Street, Suite 803
Seattle, WA 98101-1264
(800) 931-2237

Web site: http://www.nationaleatingdisorders.org
NEDA is the largest not-for-profit organization in the United
   States working to prevent eating disorders and provide
   treatment referrals to those suffering from anorexia,
   bulimia, and binge-eating, and those concerned with
   body image and weight issues.

Overeaters Anonymous (OA)
6075 Zenith Court NE
Rio Rancho, NM 87124-6424
(505) 891-4320
Web site: http://www.overeatersanonymous.org
OA is a self-help organization based on the twelve-step
   program of Alcoholics Anonymous. It offers support in
   dealing with the physical and emotional symptoms of
   compulsive eating.

Web Sites

Due to the changing nature of Internet links, Rosen
Publishing has developed an online list of Web sites
related to the subject of this book. This site is updated
regularly. Please use this link to access the list:

http://www.rosenlinks.com/msc/afnl

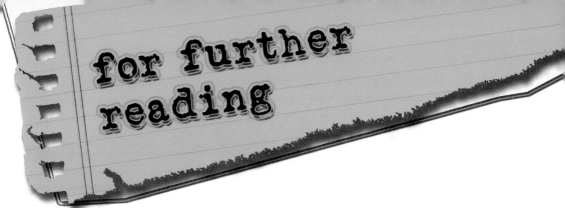

Bear, Merryl. *An Introduction to Food and Weight Problems.* Toronto, Ontario: The National Eating Disorder Information Center, 2003.

Bjorklund, Ruth. *Eating Disorders.* Tarrytown, NY: Marshall Cavendish, 2006.

Cooke, Kaz. *Real Gorgeous: The Truth About Body and Beauty.* New York, NY: W. W. Norton and Company, 1996.

Herria, Marcia. *Nancy Parent's Guide to Childhood Eating Disorders.* New York, NY: Henry Holt and Company, 2002.

Litt, Ann. *Fuel for Young Athletes.* Champaign, IL: Human Kinetics, 2004.

Loy, Spike Nasmyth and Bo Nasmyth Loy. *487 Really Cool Tips for Kids with Diabetes.* Alexandria, VA: American Diabetes Association, 2004.

McGraw, Jay. *Ultimate Weight Solution for Teens: The 7 Keys to Weight Loss Freedom.* New York, NY: Free Press, 2003.

Ruiz, Ruth Anne. *The Dangers of Binge Drinking.* New York, NY: The Rosen Publishing Group, Inc., 2000.

Salmon, Margaret Belais. *Food Facts for Teenagers: A Guide to Good Nutrition for Teens and Preteens.* Springfield, IL: Charles C. Thomas Publisher, 2002.

Sanders, Pete, and Steve Myers. *Taking Drugs* (Choices and Decisions). Mankato, MN: Aladdin Books Ltd., 2006.

Schroeder, Barbara, and Carrie Wiatt. *The Diet for Teenagers Only*. New York, NY: Regan Books, 2005.

Smith, Erica. *Anorexia Nervosa: When Food Is the Enemy*. New York, NY: The Rosen Publishing Group, 1999.

Smith, Grainne. *Anorexia and Bulimia in the Family*. Chichester, England: John Wiley & Sons, Ltd., 2004.

Vancleave, Janice. *Food and Nutrition for Every Kid*. Hoboken, NJ: John Wiley & Sons, Inc., 1999.

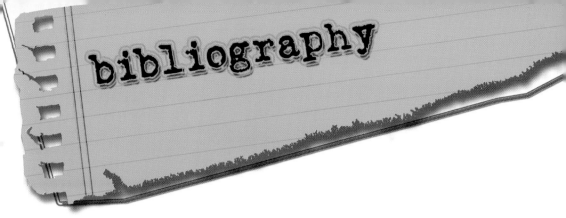

Davis, Brangien. *What's Real, What's Ideal: Overcoming a Negative Body Image.* New York, NY: The Rosen Publishing Group, 1999.

Immell, Myra H. *Eating Disorders.* San Diego, CA: Greenhaven Press, Inc., 1999.

Leone, Daniel A. *Anorexia.* San Diego, CA: Greenhaven Press, Inc., 2001.

Lynette, Rachel. *Anorexia.* Farmington Hills, MI: Kidhaven Press, 2006.

Powell, Jillian. *Food and Your Health* (Health Matters). Austin, TX: Raintree Steck-Vaughn, 1998.

Turck, Mary. *Healthy Eating for Weight Management.* Mankato, MN: Capstone Press, 2001.

Weiss Vollstadt, Elizabeth. *Teen Eating Disorders.* San Diego, CA: Lucent Books, Inc., 1999.

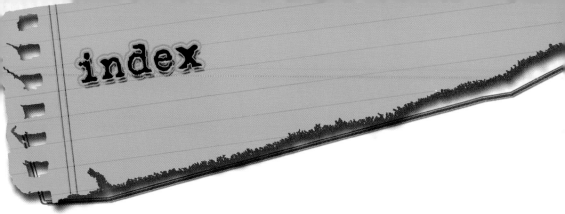

index

About the Author

Sandra Giddens has a doctorate in special education. She works with students, teachers, administrators, and parents at the Toronto District School Board as a special education consultant. Owen Giddens has a doctorate in psychology. He has worked at Toronto General Hospital treating teenagers with eating disorders. He now has a private practice where he works with children, teens, adults, individuals, and couples. Both Giddenses assist teens through their many challenges in growing up.

Photo Credits

Cover © www.istockphoto.com/Ana Blazic; p. 6 © Tony Freeman/ PhotoEdit; p. 8 © www.istockphoto.com/malcolm romain; p.10 © www.istockphoto.com/Sean Locke; p. 13 © Molly Riley/Reuters/Corbis; p. 15 © Justin Sullivan/Getty Images; p. 16 © www.istockphoto.com/Cat London; p. 18 © www.istockphoto.com/Murat Baysan; p. 20 © www. istockphoto.com/Linda Bucklin; p. 23 © www.istockphoto.com/Joseph Abbott; p. 25 © www.istockphoto.com/Barrie Holden; p. 27 © Custom Medical Stock Photo; p. 28 © Chris Hondros/Getty Images; p. 30 © Getty Images; p. 32 © www.istockphoto.com/Jim DeLillo; p. 33 (top left) © www.istockphoto.com/OlgaLIS, (top right) © www.istockphoto. com/Robyn Mackenzie, (bottom) © www.istockphoto.com/Randy Harris; p. 35 © Articulate Graphics/Custom Medical Stock Photo; p. 36 © www.istockphoto.com/Brandon Laufenberg.

Designer: Tahara Anderson; **Photo Researcher:** Amy Feinberg